REX STEVENS

A Beginners Pocketbook to Burpee Hell

A Quest for Fatigue Resistance in 30 Days with the Best Exercise You Love to Hate

First edition

This book was professionally typeset on Reedsy.
Find out more at reedsy.com

"If you are going through hell, keep going"

WINSTON CHURCHILL

Contents

1

Introduction

It is important that I put this out there now. I am a beginner and I make no bones about it. This book is written by a beginner and for beginners primarily. Does it mean that if you feel you are 'advanced' or knowledgeable in fitness you cannot glean something new from these pages? I hope you can.

Besides, what does it mean to be a beginner anyway? You can have specific expertise in one narrow aspect of fitness or perhaps your experience encompasses a broader range including all aspects of resistance training, cardio, nutrition, supplements or maybe you have a degree in kinesiology. If that is the case, this book may be too elementary for you. By same token, you may discover one nugget, one kernel of wisdom that resonates with you and if that is the case, then take it with you- and don't forget to share.

I am a beginner who had an experience, a moment, so I make no claims of being better than anyone. I am not interested in criticizing others or debating the fine points of any one exercise. There are plenty of experts out there and some true inspirations.

As cliché as it may sound: I only know my own truth and I felt compelled to share.

Like the title says- it's a beginner's journey and my truth is that the only people who do not understand the bittersweet nature of burpees are those that have not done them.

I want this to be functional for any reader but don't take risks on your health. This will be the standard line, but it is true nonetheless. You are responsible for you. Only you know your current state of health, fitness level and readiness. Check with your healthcare professional before proceeding. Do your due diligence on yourself. Do not lead with your ego- be honest about where you are at and once you do and you are good to go, read on and my hope is that in sharing you grow just bit more. In the end, growth is a game of inches.

What I will cover is my journey, the origins of burpees as well as a discussion of technique and advice on how to make the training easier [or harder] so you can adapt it to your current state.
   I will outline some of the variations of the burpee so you can understand its scope and use them accordingly over time.

This book was written as a reaction to my *personal* experience in discovering the exercise of burpees and how it affected my entire approach to my fitness goals. Although it can sound cheeky at times, I do have nothing but respect for the people that inspired me. This book is not meant to preach or to even instruct so much as it is to share. I can only hope that my writing will convey the message of exploring the possibilities in your own journey and do it with sincerity and honesty.

To all of you—those that have influenced, inspired, to those that have come before me in these experiences and those that will follow- I salute and thank you.

My Journey

My journey, if you want to call it that, began during COVID. It was during this very difficult time that I found myself, like millions of others, stuck at home and wondering how or if I would go to work? Shop? And, of course, what to do about my gym membership?

Now, I will admit here and now that, after [gleefully] canceling my gym membership, I felt a growing sense of excitement. This was the *perfect* and irrefutable, built-to-order excuse I needed to not exercise, eat copious amounts of comfort food and be able to point at the world and say "See! I just can't make it to the gym."

Little did I know that this excitement would be short lived and the sound of its death rattle would be found in the clicking of my keyboard.

It happened one evening while happily settling into a cushioned chair for yet another rabbit hole adventure on YouTube. I was presented with a thumbnail of a man in the heat of a workout. Now, normally I would not bite down on such clickbait but it was the face- glowing in the dark on my screen and drenched in sweat.

The face and the tag that did it. The face held a demonic grin and alongside this rictus were the words:

"Reps! Reps! Reps! - 750 2 Pump burpees."

My mind reeled.

I had dabbled with burpees years earlier and struggled mightily to even incorporate a dozen or so at a time in any one circuit work out. In the end, I turned away from burpees and convinced myself they did not exist; treating anyone I saw doing them like an apparition and ignoring articles that cited them as an option. They were a fitness pariah that I would not welcome into my camp under any circumstances.

750!! — This could not be.

This was unimaginable and my morbid curiosity got the better of me.

I clicked … and my dreams of blissful indolence took flight, never to return.

Forced to watch, my eyes bugged out of my head, as this monster would go on to perform, what seemed to be an endless stream of reps.

Driven, relentless- this devil spawn went on to shatter my notions on stamina and strength. He was suffering in plain sight as he pounded out hundreds of reps. Leading from the front by showing his humanity and suffering. A human locomotive that pumped out almost a thousand reps in one sitting and, in doing so, broke me and forced me to face the man in the mirror.

The message was as simple as it was honest:
Pain was inevitable but suffering was optional.
The message resonated with me.
Perhaps it was the COVID lockdown but whatever it was- it moved me.

Pain and suffering are not the same.

I heard myself citing excuses one after another 'I am too busy' 'Next week will be a fresh start' 'Just for today, I will do a partial, light workout- it's better than nothing, right?'.
Wrong-Enough was enough.

My word had to mean something and being true to it would not be easy.
Pain.
Following through would not be easy.
It would mean putting the 'grit' back in integrity.
Suffering.

That night, I committed and when I did, I knew I was hopeful but what I did not know was that...

Hell was coming.

2

Managing Expectations & The Origins of the Burpee

Managing Expectations

When I first had the idea of writing this book, I wanted it to do three things.

First, I wanted to outline a simple guide that would introduce people to the world of burpees.

Secondly, I wanted it to be short, handy and functional.

Lastly, I wanted to share some of my experiences and lessons from my own personal journey and set a simple challenge as an object lesson to kick start you on your own journey.

What Not to Expect

I believe in managing expectations so lets' get the good/bad news out of the way from the start. My promise in the upcoming pages is to be honest and authentic so here goes…

- This 30-Day Challenge is not being offered up as a cure all workout routine as much as it is a 1-time 'sample taster' meant to introduce you to burpees in all its' glory.

- It is a one-off 30-Day Challenge that focuses on burpees and should not, in my opinion, be viewed as an ongoing workout routine
- I cannot guarantee results...too much of that depends on you, I make no claims of being an expert and that is not what the book is about.
- I will not cover nutrition or supplements for the same reasons mentioned above
- I will only briefly touch on, as a matter of suggestions, cardio, lower body or pulling exercises.

What to Expect

This book is meant as an informational pocket guide and a 30-Day challenge is based on my same journey that you can choose to take...or not *[If you are reading this, I assume you are here to square your shoulders and give it a green light.]*

Along the way, I hope you do find some added value in these pages.

In the end, you will get the results you earn. You will have no one to thank or blame but yourself and that is a good thing.

It is my hope that this journey will do for you what it did for me— prove that you can, if you commit.

A Snapshot of What is Coming...

First up, I will share with you my experience The Burpee itself. Its origins, tips on technique and form along with variations and even a dash of debatable points on its merits.

Secondly, A 30-Day Challenge in the form of 6 sessions a week of burpee focused workouts. The option to add to the week up to 3 days are for you to supplement [or not] with exercises that do complement the muscles primarily targeted by burpees.

The 30- Day Challenge—is a kind preparation with some perspiration but meant as inspiration- especially for those of you with little to no experience with burpees.

It is meant to be a 'toe tester dip' into the dark waters of performing this exercise by outlining a simple and flexible 30-Day Challenge that will have you scheduling them as part of your weekly workouts.

All of this culminating with 100 Unbroken Burpees on your last day.

The Origins of the Burpee

I think most people would agree that burpees suck…

Don't get me wrong, I do burpees often and in high volume so I feel I can have an opinion on the matter.

They suck.

Every time I strap on my wrist wraps, set my tabata for time and stare down at the ground the same thought goes through my mind-"S%#t!"

There is no day you wake up screaming for joy and fist pumping when you discover burpees are on the menu for your work out.

It is what it is-burpees are more like a cold plunge than a steak dinner.

Of course, there is something to be said for embracing the suck and we will dive into that in later chapters but I feel I need to light this firecracker off by being real- so, say it with me or think it out loud-burpees suck!

They suck and that needs to be acknowledged- then set it aside forever more.

And so, like most things in life that are worthwhile- the juice is worth the squeeze.

With that said, the least asked question is who invented this bugger of an exercise that has all manner of people cringing in gyms across the world?

We have Royal H. Burpee to blame for the origins of this exercise. In my opinion, this physiologist from the 1930's had way too much time on his hands. He developed it as part of his Ph.D. thesis at Colombia University and as a full body calisthenic exercise.

It began as a simple four-count movement made up of a squat, thrusting the legs back, returning to the squat position, and standing up.

From his perspective, Royal H. Burpee saw this as an efficient and simple manner in which to evaluate the agility, coordination, and strength of individuals.

The evolution of the burpee over time included ever increasing variations meant to drive performance whilst simultaneously terrorizing those wading into the deep waters of these complex versions. The variations often include multiple 'pumps' aka push-ups; as well as incorporating the mountain climber type movements that define the notorious Navy Seal Burpee.

We will delve into these horrors in later chapters and do not be surprised if some find their way into the challenge. Regardless, Royal H. Burpee's namesake has become the best exercise we love to hate and a staple in the fitness and military communities.

3

Muscles: The What & The Why

What Muscles are you Working?

Let's talk about the basics first.

When you do a burpee, you find out quick enough that a lot of your body is engaged. It is truly a total body workout but by the same token, after only a handful of reps, you know that the 'hurt' is going to be coming.

The burpee is a simple and great way to work most major muscle groups and they can strengthen both upper and lower body. Plain and simple. A burpee is greater than the sum of its parts.

A cross fit athlete Eugene Babenko once explained that 'Twenty burpees equates to more than 20 air squats, 20 push ups and 20 jumping jacks' by 'taking the body through a full range of motion [requires] a lot of oxygen in a short period of time'

Erica Giovinazzo- a CrossFit Coach and nutritionist- further explains how burpees takes your body through various planes of motion. Unlike skipping rope or rowing where you may remain in one spot, the burpee has you moving up and down thus dramatically increasing heart rate.

It also explains the misery and commiserations it inspires among its advocates.

Burpees helps to strengthen your:

- Shoulders
- Arms
- Core
- Glutes
- Quads
- Hamstrings

Why Do Burpees?

Now in my opinion, and I think I would be supported in this, a burpee is not a cure all or the only exercise you should do. Fitness encompasses a broad spectrum and there are true professionals out there for every niche imaginable.

Having said that, as I will mention over and over again, in my experience, burpees provide a simple and efficient exercise that hits multiple muscle groups to enhance strength, stamina and cardio.

So, why do burpees? It would seem pretty obvious:

They are Just Too Damn Convenient

- If you are strapped for time?

Burpees

- If you don't have much equipment?

Burpees

- If you stuck at the office or in a hotel?

Burpees

- If you need to blow off steam or decompress?

Burpees

- If you want to spice up an existing workout?

Burpees

- If you want to target muscles by adding 'more' to chest, legs, shoulders or arms? Burpees

You get the picture.

A Special Sauce for Your Work Outs

A burpee is a calisthenic exercise. It will use your body weight for resistance. Focusing on building both lower and upper body strength and endurance through a full body work out.

Fatigue resistance does not come eary and with burpees, you will be applying yourself to an exercise that works to strengthen the muscles in your legs, hips, buttocks, abdomen, arms, chest, and shoulders.

When working on a HIIT program for example, burpees can be the *special sauce* that you can choose to add to truly spice that work out up to a thing of misery.

You can apply burpees to high intensity interval training circuits where you can use a short burst of a high intensity exercise followed by a short rest period. Burpees are made to order for this type of training when applied properly.

You will not be long into your burpees journey before you realize that when done properly and with proper pace, it is a high intensity workout sure to condition your muscle groups as well as getting your heart/lungs pumping and the sweat flowing.

Gauge Your Fitness

As Royal. H. Burpee first conceived of this crusher to effectively gauge fitness, it still remains an honest eye opener and perfect aid in measuring your ongoing fitness journey. If at some point you start feeling sore? Then it may be a strength based issue that may need to be addressed. If you are feeling winded? Then cardiovascular and stamina may need to be addressed.

Either way, burpees will be your huckleberry.

Burning Fat & Longevity

Researchers have found that doing more vigorous forms of exercise seemed to be associated with living a longer life.

Burpees will qualify as vigorous.

However, like most great workouts, technique is a centerpiece to results.

In the next chapter, we will take a closer look at the technique and variations available.

4

Technique is Everything

Technique is Important
Without supervision, it's important to talk technique. A burpee may seem pretty straightforward but there are some important fine points to keep in mind.

We will address gear such as mats, hand wraps etc. later but for the time being let's just look at the steps involved in a straightforward 1 Pump burpee.

I will be referring to the 1 Pump as the foundational single rep burpee. Here are the steps to follow:

- Standing with shoulders square and head up- Begin.
- Put your hands down in front of your feet as you squat down
- Jump your feet back as you land into a push up position
- Be sure your wrist and shoulders are in line
- Back is straight and be sure to be stable with strong core
- Perform one push up
- Use the momentum of the push up to jump back in with your feet apart [vs together]
- Stand up [Jump optional]

- Find a pace that works and repeat

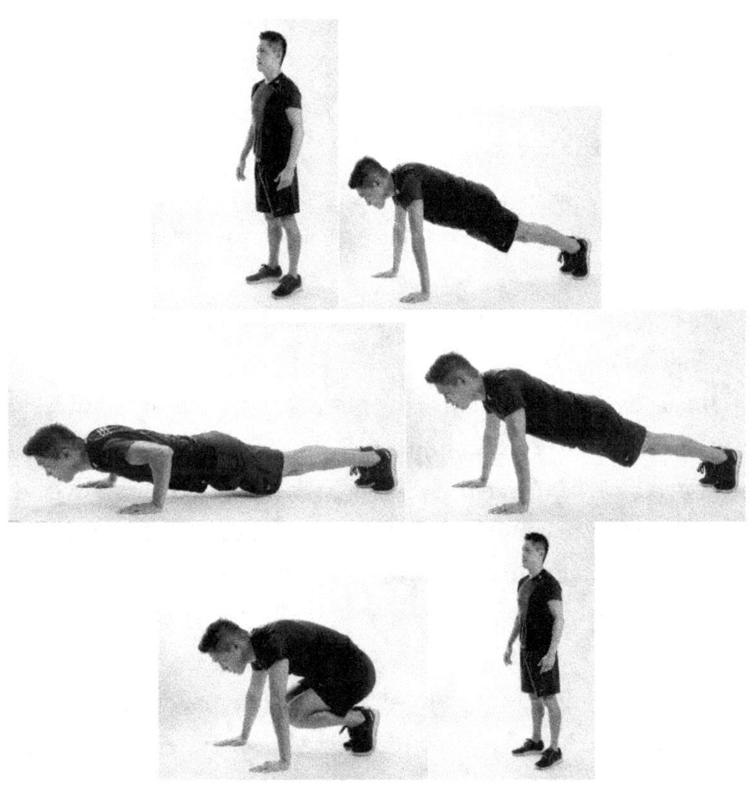

Why is Technique Important?

- *Hit the Proper Muscle Groups:* By using proper technique you will get mind-muscle connection you need to improve gains.

- *Reduce Possibility of Injury:* Well timed *and* purposeful movement will reduce chances of injury. Speed is not important but the illusion of speed will come in the form of increased pace.
- *Pace:* You will find a flow that works for you. Don't rush it and take the time you need to recover after each rep in order to perform each rep properly.

Important Mistakes to Avoid

- *Loose Core*: You have to maintain a solid, tight core during the entire exercise.
- *Dipping or Arching Back*: A sway in either direction in your back is a sign of instability
- *Hands too far ahead:* This may put a strain on your shoulders and alignment thus risking injury.
- *Jumping Back in Too Far*: Jumping back to far in in order to get back to your feet may put unnecessary pressure on your knees.
- Sacrificing technique in favor or volume is counter productive.

If you are noticing any of these signs then you may want to take note of the time, number of reps or recovery time between reps and adjust accordingly.

How to Make it Easier

If doing even one burpee is too difficult, I might suggest a few things. Firstly, don't rush it and risk injury.

Take your time and try this to get comfortable with the movement.

- *Skip the push up:* If your chest muscles or shoulders aren't ready for push ups, hold a plank position for a couple of seconds instead of doing a push up. You could also do a partial push up until you build up more strength.

- Start with a number of reps that you can manage and begin to get a feel for the movement and the effort involved. If you are like most first timers, you will wonder what you have gotten into. Once you get past that, get that number of reps out of the way then take a pause and before hitting a few more sets.
- Take stock of your baseline and you will use this in your challenge

Once you build some physical intelligence in the movement, the burpee will become increasingly simpler to execute.

As the technique becomes easier to execute you will find yourself bumping up against the next demon that you will have to face at the gates of this hell.

Volume.

But before we head to rep city where it will be truly hellish, lets take a look at some gear as well as the debate burpees have inspired among enthusiasts.

5

Gear, Yay & Nay Sayers

AWord about Gear

It is the proverbial good news/bad news.

The bad news is that you do not need any equipment to do a burpee. Sorry, no excuses to be had here! If you are short on funds? Resources or space? Drop down and hit the pavement.

The good news for you gear heads is that there are a few pieces of equipment that you can use and add to your inventory.

All are pretty inexpensive, easy to come by and I would recommend.

First, a good pair of wrist wraps. These will help increase longevity of your wrist; reduce injury and have the added bonus of making you feel pretty bad ass as you get into character to do your workout. Don't underestimate the psychological power of ripping those straps off after a successful workout - or the hesitation to do so if you are thinking of quitting-and oh! You will think about quitting- a lot!

Secondly, a rubber yoga mat will not only add some additional cushion that every part of your body will thank you for but also provide some traction. The added bonus here is that it will also prevent the sweat aplenty from seeping or pooling on your floors. Just remember to towel it off and maybe give it a squirt of vinegar and water on occasion, or it could get nasty.

By the way, a notepad and pen will come in handy if you care to keep track of your progress.

Last but not least, bring a towel and some water. Don't use it as an excuse to stop too long or take irregularly long breaks but you should re-hydrate.

The Yay and the Nay Sayers

Burpees. Funny name and dead serious exercise but there has been some debate on its merits and shortcomings. It would seem that the only thing that is unilaterally agreed upon is that no one actually likes doing them.

Here are some of the things that divide the camps.

Nay Sayers:

- Burpees put undue stress on your joints including your wrists, shoulders, knees and lower back.
- It is more of an advanced exercise, in need of higher strength and mobility which leads to higher incidence of improper form and thus lower rate of conditioning.
- The loss of form, for the reasons above, could make one prone to injury
- The only people who advocate for them are already athletic and simply enjoy doing them.
- There are better options, such as disassembling the exercise and focusing on push ups, squats and incorporating plyometrics and any cardio machine like the bike, ski erg, elliptical or simple sprints.
- In the same vein, the burpee tries to be too many things- a push

up, a plank, a squat so why not opt for a series of great tools rather than one with a lesser version of each?

- It lacks functionality in any sport specific way- no one throws themselves to the ground to get back up again.
- And last but not least- Why? Why bother with it at all. It's a silly exercise with far too many possibilities of injury, improper mechanics and it is just far better to keep it out of your routine curriculum.

The Yay Sayers:

- Undue stress on the wrists and shoulders? It is more a matter of technique than any deficiency in the exercise. If you were to do a squat jump and you land stiff legged, no one will say squat jumps are wrong, they would address your technique [and say squat jumps are fine] What about dumbbell presses? push ups? kettlebell presses? Plyometrics? It is an illogical argument.

More on this:

The burpee when done in a controlled fashion should NOT have you slamming your hands on the floor. You reach down and 'place your hands' before performing the rest of the movement.

- Mobility Issues- you cannot reach the floor? Use a raised box, platform or squat lower according to your range of motion. Problem solved.
- It's too hard or requires strength and mobility- Isn't that is the point? Isn't that training? Squat heavy-bad? Dead lift heavy-bad? Technique and strength are vital regardless of your level and good trainers find application.

- There are better options! That is subjective and compared to what? What if I am in a hotel with no exercise room? What if I am outside and have no equipment? Or I don't like running?
- People who do them just like doing them?- Yes, and people are more likely to do something they like doing- more often. Burpees are famous for the love-hate they inspire.
- In the same vein, it tries to be too many things—This argument falls apart when you look at things like Olympic lift, which can be seen as upright row, a cheat curl and shoulder press? Is it bad? What about a kettle bell swing? Is it bad because it has elements of a dead lift and a shoulder raise.
- The burpee is its own exercise and has its own identity.

All interesting points and you will make up your own mind. In the meantime, lets start to break down the challenge and like any work out there will be elements to consider.

6

The Challenge? …Wait! Reprieve!

Now that you know what burpees are; where they came from; their benefits and you even bought the gear then the time for procrastination is over. The day has arrived and you have to meet the man in the mirror. Time to do them! …

But first! [reprieve]

It's time to warm up!

Warm Up! It's a Thing.

Look, I know you are anxious to get that workout started; finish; hit a wonderful warm shower and then get on with your day but ignoring warming up is a recipe for disaster. Everyone knows it is important and yet we ignore it. Elite athletes do it and they do it every single time. Why? Because it is not optional. It's a thing and it has to be done.

So, what makes you special?

Blissfully ignorant beginners can be forgiven but now you that you have been told- or reminded-you have no excuse. Ignore warming up at your own peril.

The important thing is to get your body warm and blood flowing into those cold muscles. I am no expert but a proper warm up and cool down goes a long way in injury prevention. It also helps get you into character for what is to come.

Here are some of the warm ups I use but the internet is filled with variations.

My sequence goes as follows:

- *Neck Rolls*- gently roll your head back/forth as well as side to side and then gentle rolls around.
- *Shoulder Rolls*- pull your shoulders front, up, back and to neutral until you get a nice roll going
- *Arm Salutes*-bring your loosely straight arm up to just above your head and let them drop back and repeat with alternating arms.
- *Chain Breakers*- bring arms up with closed fists at chest and elbows locked, then open and shut arms backward while keeping elbows at chest level
- *Arm Wind Mills*- swing one arm at a time over and around to gently rotate shoulder
- *Elbow Wind Mills*- same as arm swing but swing hands around keeping elbow joint as center of the swing
- *Wrist Rolls/ Shakes*—roll wrists around the joint
- *Finger/ Wrist Bends*- using one hand on the other, gently pull your hand back on wrist to get a stretch. Repeat for both hands
- *Knee Ups* Lift one leg up toward body, bending the knee as you do, as if you were trying to touch the rib cage with knee.
- *Side Knee Swings*- Raise a bent leg and circle the leg across the body then back to ground starting position
- *Leg Kicks*- hold onto a wall or chair and swing your leg in front and back
- *Jumping Jacks*- Stand in a straight position with your feet together,

arms fully extended, hands by your sides, hop your feet out to your body's sides, swing your arms out to either side and raise them above your head and return to original position.

Alternatives can include any number of animal drill walks or simply do a few burpees.

Cool Down- the Calm after the Storm

There are a lot of stretching routines you can find online. A good cool down will help you decompress and give yourself some much-needed self-love for a job well done.

I have found that just randomly stretching has never worked as well as finding a flow that not only helps me cool down but also acts like a form of meditation in body awareness especially after a rigorous and dynamic workout. Consider it the calm after the storm.

My advice is to find a series of half a dozen or so simple post work out stretches that hit the major muscle groups in your core and legs and then put them into a sequence that you can recall and follow. I have a series that I use post workout where I start standing and end up on the ground so that I address most of my major muscle groups. I gently get into the stretch and hold each one for 30 seconds. I move on to the next posture. Once I am done, I actually start over and keep flowing through that sequence for 3-4 rounds or 10-12 minutes minimum.

Personalize it in the sense of finding a sequence that makes sense to you and feel free to shuffle them around as you move through them.

My sequence - as best as I can describe it - on the ground goes as follows:
[I recommend searching online for better description and make up your own routine]

On the ground:

1. Kneeling; my legs tucked under me and seated on my ankles- I simply sit on my ankles hands on my knees and sink slowly as far as I need to feel the stretch in my thighs.
2. Child's Pose-reach forward with your hands and drop your head down gently while keeping your backside near your ankles
3. Cat and Cow pose- move onto all fours where I raise my head, arch my back upward then drop my head into my chest and sink my shoulders with my back arched downward.
4. Go back to #1
5. Bring one leg straight back; pointed toe and bend my body over onto my bent knee
6. Bring my knee back alongside the other and repeat for alternate leg
7. Go back to #1
8. Slide off into a 50-50 S-position with one foot heel near the inside of my thigh and the other near my backside—lean forward into a stretch; even bring forehead to knee-gently.
9. Go back to #1 and repeat #8 for other leg.
10. Go back to #1 then go onto all fours and slowly get onto one leg at a time; get on your feet and roll upwards into a standing position.

Standing:

Once I am standing, I generally will follow a similar sequence of my warm up but much more gently with a focus on working out the residual tension. I skip the jumping jacks when cooling down.

Last words on warm ups and cool downs.

It's important to warm up and cool down to keep those joints and muscles ready for each workout so perform the warm ups and cool downs with the same attention to technique and control as any other workout. The tendency for some people is to get sloppy in these sections of their workout or skip them entirely. Wrong.

Respect the workout. Respect your body. Your body is a machine and subject to the same consequences of neglect.

You need to prep your body for the workout and you need to respect what your body has been through at the end of it.

Warming up as well as a proper cool down could dictate the success or failure of your experience as your body will quite or break if not cared for.

In my opinion, if you are not warming up or cooling down effectively after workouts and you are *not feeling any ill effects*, then you may not be working hard enough.

Just my 2 cents.

Now lets get into some fine points…

7

On Your Mark, Get Set…Wait!

Hold on! A few last words…

Don't Rest? Pace!

I don't mean there is no rest, but pick a pace that makes sense for you. Consider the entire set or workout and find your 'Goldilocks'.

Pro Tip:

I use a tabata app that I down loaded onto my phone. The tabata allowed me to set the duration of an exercise. The duration of an exercise, in my routines, was the time allotted to me to perform 1 Rep. So, get a sense of how long it takes you to do 1 Rep, then add on the recovery time you need before performing another rep and that total is the pace you are going to use.

Finder your inner 'Goldilocks'

Finding the proper pace will not only help you get into a flow state, but in finding it you will have a diagnostic tool at your disposal that informs you of what your body can handle. You may also want to look at the demands of the entire workout and adjust accordingly.

- If you are going to 'hot'- you will burn out; take too many breaks or worse-quit.
- If you are going to 'cool'- you are not working hard enough and that defeats the purpose of working out.
- If you find the *sweet spot*- you will feel the burn, but be able to keep repping.

Find a pace that is comfortably uncomfortable. Get the idea?

Breathe

As crazy as it sounds- remember to breathe. Having said that, you may find that a pattern emerges. The pattern I found is inline with a 6 count as this 1 Pump is often referred to:

- Inhale standing
- Exhale into squat and hand placement
- Inhale with legs shoot out and
- Exhale as I lower into the push up
- Inhale as I raise up in the push up and leg jump recovery and
- Exhale to stand.

Regardless of your pacing, get into a rhythm and keep steady.

Feet and Hand Coordination

You will find that over time, your coordination of hand placement in conjunction with shooting your feet out will become smoother and more graceful. In fact, you may notice that there will come a time when your hands are actually landing *before* your feet do. This is a 'hand before feet moment' and should not be rushed or aimed for particularly.

Just be aware of your body moving fluidly through the motion and the awareness will come on its own.

Core Intact & Eyes Forward

Keep your core intact, eyes forward throughout with the integrity of body alignment intact.

Beast Mode

When you start working out with burpees you will find it is a uniquely solitary exercise. You may begin by paying attention to each element of dropping to the floor, feet back, push up and jump into standing until you have that flow. However, a time will have to come when you hit auto pilot and just GO! And GO! And GO!

This is where you are going to get into the zone and start finding out about yourself.

You will hit a wall. Sometimes the wall will win and other times you may tuck your shirt in and get into beast mode and go a few reps more.

Beast mode gets down to going one more time. One reps builds on another- the pain is inevitable but the suffering is optional. You can only learn this lesson the hard way.

Trust me.

A Few Storms to Prep for the Hurricane

Some prep work can go a long way.

Before the 30-Day Challenge it may be in your interest to prep with a variety of exercises centered on burpees. What follows is a short list of some variations.

You do not have to do all these or any of them to be honest. What I would have you do is pick one [or a few] and grind them it into your existing workouts.

Again, if you not presently working out, then fashion workouts that are light and easy over the week[s] prior to your challenge month that hit all body parts of your upper, lower body, throw in some cardio and remember to warm up and cool down.

You need to get some physical intelligence back into your system and nervous system as a sort of wake-up call for what is about to come.

My go to is #2 with a few twists.

I perform a burpee with a series of 'pumps' meaning push ups. A 2-Pump is a burpee with 2 push ups built into the lower phase before jumping back to your feet.

A 3-Pump is a burpee with 3 push ups built into it and so on.

You get the idea. I have integrated 1,2,3 up to 9 and 10 pumps into workouts over the years and the more time you spend in the lower phase the greater the tax you pay with muscle strength and stamina.

Variety is the Spice of Life

Here are the variations on the theme of burpees that not only serve to challenge you on your journey but will add the kind of variety that would make the Marquis de Sade quail.

Most of these will not be involved with the challenge but it gives you a sense of the scope and flexibility you can have in performing burpees.

This list is by no means complete and once you begin to do your own research you will find endless variations.

For your sweat popping consideration here are 10 Burpee exercise routines designed to build strength and cardiovascular endurance.

Each routine will target different muscle groups and add variety to your workouts.

Important:

Keep in mind the sets and reps cited are strictly meant as guidelines— feel free to play with the number of sets and reps

Here you go:

1. **Standard Burpees**

   - Perform standard Burpees for 3 sets of 15 reps. Rest for 60 seconds between sets.

2. **Burpee with Push-Up**

- Perform a Burpee with a push-up at the plank position. Complete 3 sets of 12 reps. Rest for 60 seconds between sets.

These Burpee Push-Ups are my go-to in almost every workout. In time and certainly in the challenge you will be pushed to apply 2 pumps [aka 2 push ups] or 3 pumps and onward to each burpee. I have gone as far as having 10 pumps in a burpee routine and I can assure you the pumps will add a level of activation that is something else.

3. **Burpee Box Jumps**

- After performing the squat and plank portion of the Burpee, jump onto a sturdy box or bench instead of jumping straight up. Do 3 sets of 10 reps. Rest for 90 seconds between sets.

4. **Burpee with Tuck Jump**

- After returning to the standing position, perform a tuck jump by bringing your knees to your chest as you jump. Perform 3 sets of 12 reps. Rest for 60 seconds between sets.

5. **Burpee with Mountain Climbers**

- After reaching the plank position, perform 4 mountain climbers (2 per leg) before jumping back to the squat position. Do 3 sets of 10 reps. Rest for 60 seconds between sets.

6. **Burpee to Pull-Up**

- Perform a Burpee under a pull-up bar. After the jump, grab the bar and do a pull-up. Complete 3 sets of 8 reps. Rest for 90 seconds between sets.

7. **Burpee with Dumbbell Press**

- Hold a pair of light dumbbells. After the push-up, as you jump back to standing, press the dumbbells overhead. Perform 3 sets of 10 reps. Rest for 60 seconds between sets.

8. **Single-Leg Burpees**

- Perform the Burpee on one leg, alternating legs each rep. Do 3 sets of 10 reps per leg. Rest for 60 seconds between sets.

9. **Burpee with Plank Jack**

- In the plank position, perform a plank jack by jumping your feet wide apart and back together before completing the Burpee. Do 3 sets of 12 reps. Rest for 60 seconds between sets.

Note: When you combine a push up into this, it will be referred to as a Body Builder Burpee

10. **Burpee AMRAP (As Many Reps as Possible) **

- Set a timer for 5 minutes and perform as many Burpees as possible within the time frame. Focus on maintaining good form and pace yourself.

All of these are morbidly fascinating and I have used many of them but as I have mentioned earlier, a burpee is not a magic pill and in the next chapter I will speak both the challenge for 30 days as well as my first time doing 500 1 pump burpee in a session.

8

Challenge Details & My 1st 500

A **Workout to be Adapted**

The challenge in the last chapters is a 30-day workout – *kind of...*

- If you presently do not have a 3-day workout, you are going to have to get one.
- If you presently work out 3 or 6 day a week then bravo.

Either way, the challenge is to go 6 days a week of burpee hell as outlined and to keep some of your present workouts while removing others.

The last day of the challenge will be to perform 100 burpees unbroken.

[The term 'Unbroken' does not mean without rest, it means choosing a pace and sticking to it during the entire set]

Burpees & The Need for Balance in All Things

Burpees is not a magic pill.

It should not and cannot be the only exercise you utilize in workouts.

Why?

Burpees is hybrid like exercise-it, like any other, is not meant to be the only exercise you do. If you want balance in your fitness and more importantly if you want to avoid injury then you need to address the needs of your whole body.

As a matter of fact, if you are serious, you should be anxious to do some homework and research in finding other exercises to incorporate into the challenge outlined in the end of this book.

You may or may not already have some experience and this process is as good a way to start as any. Just keep in mind, that with burpees are not a one stop shop and it is important to balance them out with exercises that address its' blind spots.

Which to keep and Which to Replace

Burpees, although a hybrid exercise can be seen as targeting 'pushing' muscles so balancing that requires some attention to the 'pulling' muscles and the posterior chain in general. Lower body, although taxed are larger muscle groups and can handle some added volume.

My suggestion is you can make one of two choices:

1. Do the challenge as it stands for 30 days and add no other workouts.
2. Do the challenge as it stands and blend in some added workouts [up to 3] on the days of your choice that target 'pulling', lower body, core muscle groups or cardio.

For example:

- Lower body such as air squats, lunges, calf raises, maybe even some plyometrics
- Posterior chain such as pull ups [assisted if need be], chin ups, rows etc.
- Core work such as leg raises, flutter kicks, ab rollers etc. as well as

- Cardio such as skipping, running, swimming, cycling etc.

Add these alternatives up to 3 times into your full week of burpees and let the burpees target the pushing aspect of your workouts.

Leaving my Ego at the Door: The Hare & the Tortoise

Ultimately, try to stay on course for the 30-Day Challenge but listen to your body.

If you feel the added workouts you are doing besides the burpees are burning you out, then subtract some of them. Working out in any manner 6 days a week can be taxing.

As you progress, as your strength increases and ligaments and joints adapt you may find yourself increasing the volume of burpees in the future but if you are have not done burpees in any serious form before, there will be an adaption period so:

- Be patient-don't rush through the movement, ever.
- Pace yourself- I adjusted the timer for any one rep on my tabata phone app exercise to find my sweet spot. The 'exercise' duration allowed me to both perform the exercise and still recover before performing the next rep.
- Adjust the Pace- check your ego and adjust your pace to find your flow.

If you recall the proverbial story of the race between the tortoise and the hare, then you will get the message.

I was more like the hare when I first began and I quickly realized I could not keep the pace. I was winded, burning out and viewing the entire work out as absolutely impossible. It was hell and I felt demoralized and thought of quitting…again.

However, once I adjusted my pace which allowed me to catch my breath, I began to fall into a flow. The workout got completed, and more importantly I learned a lesson that not only helped me push me to my true limits but I also realized I had an added metric to measure my progress.

My 1ˢᵗ 500

In my experience I started out struggling to squeeze out 10 reps unbroken so the idea of knocking out 20, 30 much less hundreds was out of my realm of experience. So, it was not burpees every day in volume. Some days were strictly burpee based and with significant increasing levels of volume but alternate days were meant to balance things out with workouts that targeted other large muscle groups such as legs or core. There were days that targeted legs with a mix of air squats and lunges and others that focused on pulling exercises for my back such as pull ups and chin ups and even used varied wide and narrow grips.

Assisted Pulls:

Did I mention assisted pull ups and chin ups?

If not, I will say it again- I used assisted pull ups and chin ups. The rubber bands available for that allowed me to blend pulls into my routines—and what a difference it made to my progress.

Again, I started with 1 single rep and was able to build on that double digit reps—

but that is a book for another day.

I also added mountain climbers and core exercises such as leg raises, flutter kicks and hello dollies. Some days were a kitchen sink mix of everything including burpees.

Oh, and I ran…and I hate running, but that will be the subject of another kind of hell I had to endure.

I remained true to my workouts each and every day.

The result? On the last day of my first month I completed 500 1 pump burpees in a single session.

It was ugly.

I wanted to quit every step of the way. I cursed, I spat, I groaned and I cried out for my mama. I may even have shed a few tears- but it would have been hard to tell with the pool of sweat that lay at my feet and drenched my entire t shirt, shorts and socks.

I made the mistakes. An error in my Golilocks moment had me jack rabbiting at a tempo that was far too fast, and I hit the wall way too early and I hit it HARD.

You don't know what you don't know and I had never faced this kind of volume.

I was sucking air and I felt a burn creeping up on me that stopped me in my tracks.

Yes, I stopped but only for a minute in order to get my head right and choose a pace I knew would give me a fighting chance.

I took a deep breath, looked up then down and went for it.

Almost 2 hours later it was done!

And, and all I could do was raise my fist in the air. It felt amazing.

The Lesson Learned

Now, you may not think 500 is much of an accomplishment. Perhaps you are a burpee machine and have knocked out hundreds or even thousands of burpees in your time. I applaud you, truly I do. However, for me, that day and at my age- it was a turning point and it brought me to this point where I wanted to share that experience with anyone who could relate to emotion of feeling limited.

I never thought I could, but I did. It wasn't a miracle; a fluke or a one off. Looking back, I realize it was, if I had to be honest, a product of disgust. I was disgusted with the version of myself that watched while other took action in achieving fitness goals. I am not talking about making the Olympics I mean just getting in shape, whatever that shape was that you aspired to.

Funny thing is that I am not that guy in most aspects of my life. As a matter of fact, I had a pretty successful career and personal life but when it came to working out, I turned away or quit on pushing myself far too often for my liking. I lied to myself one too many times and it came to a tipping point.

I decided no more and I committed to those 30 days. I dedicated myself in that month to being the best version of myself.

I gave my word to myself- and my word had to mean something.

Discipline, dedication, consistency of effort and integrity were my mantras during the workouts themselves. I remember repeating the phrase "Who you gonna be today!" – and I said it out loud to check myself back into character.

Yes, people have done far more reps in less time and I am certainly still a work in progress but I felt something. It was my personal moment- and I hope this simple challenge sets you on the road to finding yours.

Now, there two types of people that may be reading this right now.

One type has already had that moment and bought this book simply looking for some information on burpees, perhaps a few added insights or variations that they can add to their existing routines. For that person, I really do hope you find at least one pearl here to take with you. If not, apologies.

The second type, may still have not had that burpee moment and if anything within these pages helps you find it- with or without the 30-Day Challenge- then mission accomplished.

Let Me just Stop and Add this...

At the start of this book, I promised I would be honest.

Having just read these past few paragraphs over I realize that I have been less than honest or - maybe just not honest enough.

I did *not stay true to my workouts*- I fell short on more than a few occasions.

I missed a few workouts and had to shrink and skip a few sets or tapper down a few reps to get through a session.

I have to come clean. I have to own those lesser versions of myself if I am going to take any measure of credit in completing 500.

Looking back, they were more than a few moments of weakness. I looked myself in the mirror, more often than I care to admit, and ripped myself a new one for a piss poor performance that was not worthy of the image I was aspiring to. I reminded myself of who I was, where I came from and where I was headed. I forced myself to acknowledge my weakness and failed performance- and, although I accepted it as part of the process, I promised myself that I would push myself.

Yes, I did checked myself and I adapted but most importantly I forgave myself then I moved on.

Lastly, I asked myself to recommit to the 30-day cycle on a day to day basis.

I literally asked myself out loud and I needed to hear that answer out loud.

Looking back, that was the key. I recommitted.

- Did I fall short on occasion as I mentioned? YES, I DID.
- Did life get in the way randomly? YES, IT DID.
- Did I think about quitting every single morning of every single day? YES I DID.

But

- Did I quit? NO.

Do & Don't Do

What you don't do is sometimes more important than what you do.

And, in the end, that was the true lesson. The act of not quitting rewarded me with that amazing feeling of success. I felt like more. It provided me with a touchstone of what I was capable of if I did one thing- if I did not quit. Sounds pretty obvious and you might say that the notion of not quitting is kind of baked into the cake of committing, yes? But it is really just turning the concept on its side- of seeing both sides of the same coin needed to succeed.

Do and Don't do.

Maybe by sharing on a personal note, it may ring clearer for you.

For a long time, I would say to myself:

"I did do 500 burpees!" – and it felt great.

But the day I said: "I did 500 burpees and did not quit!"- it put lump in my throat.

It was emotional.

And looking back, I think that is when I realized that I wanted to share that horrible experience with others. Misery may love company but that kind of hell has room for all of us and going through it, for me, was something I needed to share.

This is the real motivation behind writing this book and I hope the message is getting clearer.

Find your moment, if it is noct this challenge, then find another.

Find something to challenge yourself with. Put it in your head, feel it in your heart that you need to find it and it will come. It will present itself to you. In my case, it came in the form of a simple YouTube video that made me face myself and forced me to take action.

It will not be easy and it may mean wading through your own hellish waters, but that journey is yours to take. Do or don't do.

Burpees. A silly thing with a silly name.
Who would have thought.

9

The 30-Day Challenge

F inally, after all of this, here we go.

At the risk of sounding redundant, the point of the challenge on the surface may seem to 'get into shape' and that would be fair to say but I would argue that the spirit of the challenge is to commit, to discipline yourself on principle to an idea or goal.

On the other hand, the challenge is optional. You are under no obligation to do it, if after reading these pages you feel like the timing is not right. You can do it now, delay it or toss it out altogether. It is your choice.

Building fatigue resistance with burpees takes time but once you begin to adapt and integrate them into pre-existing routines or ones that you have fashioned yourself, the results will speak for themselves.

Beginner? Intermediate? Advanced?

Although I have fashioned this for what I would deem beginners, there are far too many variables to control for at arms-length to accurately gauge anyone's level of readiness. Besides, the obvious differences in age, gender, physical health or past injuries there are flexibility, mobility issues and the list goes on. A true assessment in person by a professional would be ideal but, in the absence that, here a few more suggestions.

If, once you review the work out or after you are a few days into it, you feel it is beyond you-then you have two choices. First check your ego, then...

You can scale back the sets or reps in hopes that your progress over the month will allow you to complete the challenge or...

You can pause the challenge to address your readiness. Take the experience as a diagnostic tool that allows you to identify your weak points then let it inform your workout schedule then to take another run at it.

If you are more experienced with a level of fitness that you feel can justify increasing the demands then you can scale the reps and sets up accordingly.

How can we get a thumbnail estimate on your level?

The 3 Minute Timer Test

A simple quick test may be to do a 3-minute timer where you perform as many burpees as you can. The number of reps will give you a sense of how to scale accordingly. In rough terms a beginner may be in the 10-20 range, a strong intermediate may hit 30 and an elite may hit as much as 50. Age, gender and physical impingements aside.

Besides this 3 Min Test, you will have a sense after your first few work outs.

Technique Not the Clock

The focus should be on proper form and not on the clock. I cannot stress enough the importance of approaching this or any challenge with humility. An attitude of doing what you can and then squeezing out 1 or 2% more will take you farther than leading with your ego and quitting half way through.

If you feel tired that is normal. If you feel pain, in your joints or ligaments etc.- then stop and evaluate.

No one knows your body better than you.

With that said, here you go.

Perform the 30-Day Challenge below over any 30-day period.

Be sure to take your rest day to recover, rehydrate, stretch.

The alternate days I would recommend a suitable added workout that can include:

- Pull Ups, chin ups, rows
- Air squats, lunges
- Core exercises, Dips
- Cardio

Types of Exercises and Workouts

During the month there are types of burpees and workouts:

- **Multiple Pumps**-The 1,2 and 3 Pump burpees are performed with 1,2 or 3 push ups in the lower phase of the movement before getting back to your feet.
- **A Body Builder Burpee**- this variation has you, having done a push up and while still in the lowered position, in a plank position with arms extended, you jump your feet past shoulder width and jump them back again to shoulder width. Complete the movement and get to your feet. This should resemble hopping on your toes

outward and back into your plank with arms extended.

- **A Navy Seal Burpee**- this variation has you down in plank position and after completing your first push up, you lifting your foot to bring one knee up towards your chest then bring your knee back with both feet back on the floor. Repeat for each knee. Once both knees have been kneed up, then you complete the movement back up to your feet. This should resemble a mountain climber movement with each knee up separated by a push up.

- **A Ladder Routine**- this is a routine that is either ascending or descending in reps. For example, a 1-10 Ladder is a workout where you perform 1rep; rest; perform 2 reps at pace then 3 reps at pace until you reach 10 reps performed in succession at pace. A descending is the same principal except you begin with 10 reps and scale downward to 1 rep to complete.

- **Timed Exercise**- a timed exercise is performed for the maximum number of reps you can manage in the allotted time. You don't have to follow a pace or set number of breaks. You are competing with the clock and it is not only a nutcracker but taps your mental strength. It's a sprint that seems to go on forever. Again, take note, it will give you a good assessment of you progress.

Pace- Again? It can make you or break you!

Pick a tempo that feels comfortably uncomfortable for you and one that you may adjust during the workout.

You may find that the pace at the start of the month, is not the same as the one at the end. As a matter of fact, certain variations may demand different tempos.

In some cases, you may need to take a break during a set—and, especially in the early phases of the challenge, that may be bound to happen.

During the month, you may be in the tail end of a workout and you realize you need a bit more time to recover.

The important thing is to differentiate between catching your breath and avoidance.

Just don't quit. While completing my first 500 rep session, my pace changed multiple times and I did need to take few breathers but it got done.

Over time, my stamina and fatigue resistance grew and I went on to do 100, 200, even 250 burpees on pace. I am presently working on completing my first 500 unbroken.

And that brings me to your first 100.

100 Unbroken

The last day of the challenge is 100 Burpees unbroken.

Again, unbroken does not mean there is no rest, it means you choose a pace that makes sense to you and one that you can maintain throughout the exercise.

If you use a tabata app on your phone, you can set the exercise interval to say, 15 seconds, which means you have time to perform the exercise and you should still have time to recover slightly before the signal to exercise. The cycles or reps should be set to 100 reps.

Now, if you need to pick 20 seconds or even 25 seconds, so be it- just maintain the pace.

A typical 1 pump burpee is often called a 6 Count, and as the name suggests, it is about 6 seconds to complete.

In my opinion, anyone doing 100 reps at sub 10 seconds is advanced/ elite. As a beginner you may double that at 20 seconds, so just find your groove. By the 30th day you should have a pretty good sense of the timing.

Let us move on to the workout itself.

30 Day Challenge Work Outs

Week 1

- Monday- 1-Pump Burpee: 10 Sets of 5 Reps
- Tuesday- 1-Pump Burpee: 5 Sets of 10 Reps
- Wednesday- Ascending Ladder of 1-Pump Burpee: 1 to 10 Reps
- Thursday- 1-Pump Burpee: 10 Sets of 5 Reps
- Friday- 1-Pump Burpee: 5 Sets of 10 Reps
- Saturday- 1-Pump Burpee: Timed 12 Min Max Reps
- Sunday- Rest, Relax & Stretch

Week 2

- Monday- 2-Pump Burpee: 10 Sets of 5 Reps
- Tuesday- Descending Ladder of Body Builders: 10 to 1 Reps
- Wednesday- 2-Pump Burpee: 5 Sets of 10 Reps
- Thursday- Ascending Ladder of Navy Seals: 1 to 10 Reps
- Friday- 3-Pump Burpee: 10 Sets of 5 Reps
- Saturday- 1-Pump Burpee: Timed 12 Min Max Reps
- Sunday- Rest, Relax & Stretch

Week 3

- Monday- [2 Rounds] 5 Sets of 5 Reps:

with [Sets: 1ˢᵗ 3 Pumps/2ⁿᵈ 2 Pumps/ 3ʳᵈ Navy Seals/ 4ᵗʰ Body Builders/ 5ᵗʰ 1 Pump]

- Tuesday- Descending Ladder of 2 Pump Burpee: 10 to 1 Reps
- Wednesday- 5 Sets of 10 Reps:

with [Sets: 1ˢᵗ 2 Pumps/ 2ⁿᵈ Body Builders/ 3ʳᵈ 3 Pump/ 4ᵗʰ Navy Seals/ 5ᵗʰ 1 Pump]

- Thursday- Ascending Ladder of Body Builders: 1 to 10 Reps

with 2 Rounds of 1-Pump Burpee for 10 Reps as Finisher

- Friday- 2 Pump Burpee: 10 Sets of 5 Reps

with 2 Rounds of 1- Pump Burpee 10 Rep as Finisher

- Saturday- 1-Pump Burpee: Timed 12 Min Max Reps
- Sunday- Rest, Relax & Stretch

Week 4

- Monday- Navy Seals: 10 Sets of 5 Reps
- Tuesday- 5 Sets of 10 Reps

with [Sets: 1ˢᵗ 2 Pump/ 2ⁿᵈ Body Builders/ 3ʳᵈ 3 Pump/ 4ᵗʰ Navy Seals/ 5ᵗʰ 1 Pump]

- Wednesday- 3 Rounds of Descending Ladder of 5 to 1

with [Sets: 1st Navy Seals/ 2nd 3 Pump / 3rd 3 Body Builder / 4th 2 Pump / 5th 1 Pump]

- Thursday- Ascending Ladder of 2 Pump Burpee

with 5 Rounds of 1 Pump Burpee of 5 Reps [within 1 min per round]

- Friday- Rest/Relax
- Saturday- 1 Pump Burpees: **1 Set of 100 Reps: Unbroken**
- Sunday- Rest, Relax & Stretch

Congratulations!

If you completed the challenge, then take a minute and let it feel good.

I am sure you began the challenge with some doubt and some degree of trepidation and that would make you normal.

It is normal to have doubts or perhaps even think it an impossibility to complete 100 reps in succession…but you did. And so, if that impossibility is now possible to you, then perhaps there are other limitations worth exploring and challenging yourself with.

I wish you luck and only the best in that journey.

Peace.

10

Conclusion

I n closing, I hope you have enjoyed reading this book as much as I have enjoyed writing it.

As a pocketbook, it was meant to be informative and functional and perhaps on some level inspirational. As a handbook, I hope you will reference it on your own journey.

As a final word, I would like to say that if you feel that there was some value to be had in these pages, feel free to pass it forward.

Lastly, I would be very appreciative *if you left a favorable review on Amazon!*

Peace

11

References & Citations

Research Trusted Source

Heydari, M., Freund, J., & Boutcher, S. H. (2012). The effect of High-Intensity Intermittent exercise on body composition of overweight young males. *Journal of Obesity, 2012,* 1–8. https://doi.or g/10.1155/2012/480467

https://www.ncbi.nlm.nih.gov/pmc/articles/PMC3375095/

Research Trusted Source

Effect of moderate to vigorous physical activity on All-Cause mortality in middle-aged and older Australians. (2015, June). National Center for Biotechology Information.

Retrieved June 3, 2024, from https://pubmed.ncbi.nlm.nih.gov/2584 4882/

Gebel, K., Ding, D., Chey, T., Stamatakis, E., Brown, W. J., & Bauman, A. E. (2015). Effect of moderate to vigorous physical activity on All-Cause mortality in middle-aged and older Australians. *JAMA Internal Medicine, 175*(6), 970. https://doi.org/10.1001/jamainternmed.2015.0541

Podstawski, R., Markowski, P., Clark, C. T., Choszcz, D., & Gronek, P. (2019, October). *International standards for the 3-Minute Burpee*

Test: High- intensity motor performance. National Library of Medicine. Retrieved June 3, 2024, from https://www.ncbi.nlm.nih.gov/pmc/artic les/PMC6815084/#:~:text=The%20results%20were%20expressed%20 on,best%20female%20participant%20–%2073%20burpees

Weight Loss: Common Mistakes You Should Avoid While Performing Burpees. (2021, June 2). NTV.com. https://www.ndtv.com/health/weight-loss-common-mistakes-you -should-avoid-while-performing-burpees-2451540

Cronkleton, E. (2019, January 25). *Bodyweight exercise routines for beginners and more advanced.* Healthline.com. **https://www.healthline.com/health/bodyweight-workout** *To burpee or not to burpee.* (n.d.). Retrieved June 3, 2024, from https://a thletesacceleration.com/author/admin/

LAGIMODIERE, D. (2016, January 28). *The 3-minute burpee challenge.* Men's Health. Retrieved June 3, 2024, from https://www.menshealth.c om/uk/fitness/a749868/the-3-minute-burpee-challenge/ https://www.menshealth.com/uk/fitness/a749868/the-3-minute- burpee-challenge/

7 REASONS YOU SHOULD DO BURPEES EVERY DAY. (n.d.-b). live-fit.com. Retrieved June 3, 2024, from https://livefit.com/blogs/livefit/ 7-reasons-you-should-do-burpees-every-day#:~:text=Because%20bur pees%20target%20so%20many,move%20better%20and%20feel%20bett er. Walsh, M. (n.d.). *Use these exercises to improve your warm up routine.* Exante. Lebow, I. (n.d.). *How to do the perfect burpee (C'mon, you know you want to).* greatist.com. Retrieved June 3, 2024, from https://greatist.com/fitn

ess/how-to-do-the-perfect-burpee#tl-dr

Roland, J. (2019, September 18). *The Benefits of Burpees and How to Do Them*. Healthline.com. Retrieved June 3, 2024, from https://www.heal thline.com/health/how-to-do-a-burpee#takeaway

Coles, R. (2019, October 1). *Legal Disclaimer Examples for Books*. Cascadia Author Services. Retrieved June 3, 2024, from https://cas cadiaauthorservices.com/legal-disclaimer-examples-for-books/

Tumminello, N. (2019, March 14). *The Gorilla Burpee* [Video]. YouTube. Retrieved June 3, 2024, from https://www.youtube.com/watch?v=LN C8QZ-NKHc

Shvartsburg, A. (2020, April 10). *Nutrition, Programming Burpees, Supplements and Form, Let's talk about it* [Video]. Youtube. Retrieved June 3, 2024, from https://www.youtube.com/watch?v=c6R9LKJZxAQ

Shvartsburg, A. (2020b, May 21). *Discipline,Leadership, and Crushing Goals* [Video]. Youtube. Retrieved June 3, 2024, from https://www.you tube.com/watch?v=wxLMebEJUXU

Shvartsburg, A. (2021, April 21). *The Only Routine You Need — (750 2 pump burpees)* [Video]. Youtube. Retrieved June 3, 2024, from https://w ww.youtube.com/watch?v=vSKE304LJII